FLEXIBILITY WORKOUTS FOR WOMEN OVER 50

Daily Exercise for Seniors to lose Weight, build core strength, Enhance balance, Mobility and Achieve Good Health

Jacqueline R. Jensen

TABLE OF CONTENT

INTRODUCTION

In a world where the pressures of everyday life sometimes dictate sedentary habits, Jane's journey serves as a painful warning of the serious consequences of disregarding one's physical well-being.

 For years, Jane was stuck in a pattern that focused around lengthy periods of sitting, whether at her desk, on her commute, or relaxing in front of the television at the end of the day.

As the years went by, this lifestyle took its toll, resulting in a slew of health conditions that gradually sapped her vigor and passion for living.

Despite periodic attempts to include exercise into her schedule, Jane constantly prioritized other responsibilities before her personal health. Ignoring the continual murmurs of pain emerging from her joints and the growing sensation of weakness pervading her body, she pushed through each day, accepting that she simply lacked the time or energy to address these problems.

It wasn't until a particularly terrible bout of joint pain rendered her immobile and acutely aware of the constraints imposed by her neglected physical condition that Jane decided something needed to happen.

Faced with the sobering truth of her worsening health, she set out on a quest for answers, determined to retake control of her well-being and bring energy back into her life.

Enter "Flexibility Workouts for Women Over 50," a light of hope on Jane's path to rejuvenation. Within its pages, she discovered not only a detailed guide to recovering flexibility and strength, but also a road map for establishing a long-term commitment to wellbeing that went beyond physical activity. Written with sensitivity and competence, the book was a reliable companion on Jane's journey to recovery, providing practical techniques adapted to the specific needs of women navigating the complications of aging.

Jane set off on her road to holistic well-being, armed with new information and a renewed sense of purpose. With each gentle stretch and mindful movement, she progressively recovered control of her body, creating resilience and vigor where there was before just stagnation.

Jane emerged from her health issues stronger, more vibrant, and immeasurably thankful for the gift of fresh energy, fueled by the transformational force of her own determination and the instruction provided by "Flexibility Workouts for Women Over 50."

Today, Jane exemplifies the strength of resilience and the tremendous impact of prioritizing self-care. Her story is an example to women worldwide, a reminder that it is never too late to start on the path to wellness, and that transformation is not only possible, but inevitable, with effort, support, and a desire to accept change.

Chapter 1: Importance of Flexibility in Aging Bodies

Flexibility is essential for preserving general health and mobility, particularly as our bodies age. As women approach the age of 50 and beyond, addressing flexibility becomes increasingly vital to combat the natural reduction in muscle mass and joint function.

Incorporating flexibility exercises into their regimen can help reduce the symptoms of aging and increase quality of life.

One of the most important benefits of flexibility exercises for women over 50 is the preservation of joint mobility. As we age, our joints stiffen owing to decreased synovial fluid production and cartilage wear and tear.

Flexibility activities, such as yoga, Pilates, and stretching regimens, can help maintain or enhance joint range of motion, lowering the likelihood of stiffness and discomfort.

Flexibility exercise helps improve posture and balance, both of which are critical for avoiding falls and retaining independence. Women's posture may vary as they age, due to factors such as weakening core muscles and decreasing bone density.

Regular flexibility exercises can help strengthen the muscles that maintain normal posture and enhance balance, lowering the risk of falls and related injuries.

Flexibility exercises are also important for minimizing muscular stress and the risk of injury. Tight muscles can cause discomfort and increase the risk of strains and sprains, particularly during physical activity or regular jobs.

Stretching and flexibility exercises can assist women over 50 relieve muscular tension, enhance circulation, and promote relaxation.

Flexibility exercise may improve both physical and emotional health. Many flexibility exercises, such as yoga and tai chi, include mindfulness and relaxation methods, which can help decrease stress, improve mood, and improve overall quality of life.

Flexibility is essential for women's health and movement as they age, especially those over fifty. Women who incorporate flexibility activities into their routines can maintain joint mobility, improve posture and balance, relieve muscular stress, and increase mental health.

Prioritizing flexibility is a proactive step in aging gracefully and maintaining independence and energy in later life.

Realistic Goal Setting

Realistic goal setting is essential for women over 50 who are starting flexibility training. Setting attainable goals promotes growth while reducing the danger of injury or burnout. Here's a detailed way to set realistic goals for flexibility exercises:

Assess your current flexibility level. This might include easy tests such as touching your toes or reaching for your heels. Understanding where you're starting gives a foundation for creating reasonable goals.

Identify Areas for Improvement: Identify particular areas where you wish to increase flexibility. Women over 50 often focus the back, hips, shoulders, and hamstrings. By concentrating on these areas, you may personalize your goals to meet your own needs.

Set SMART goals: To frame your goals, use the S.M.A.R.T. criteria: specific, measurable, attainable, relevant, and time-bound. Instead of "improve flexibility," set a target such as "increase hamstring flexibility by 2 inches within 8 weeks."

Gradual Progression: Resist the urge to establish unrealistic goals that may lead to frustration or harm. Instead, favor incremental improvement. Begin with simpler, more manageable objectives, then gradually increase the intensity or duration of your exercises as your flexibility improves.

Listen to Your Body: Flexibility exercises should never cause discomfort. Be aware of your body's signals and alter your goals accordingly. If you experience any pain or resistance, change your strategy or see a competent fitness specialist.

Incorporate range: Keep your flexibility workouts interesting by using a range of exercises and approaches. This not only minimizes boredom, but also guarantees that you target diverse muscle groups and movement patterns for overall flexibility improvement.

Track Your Progress: Monitor your progress on a regular basis to keep motivated and accountable. This might include maintaining a workout log, collecting measurements, or utilizing fitness monitoring apps.

Recognize and appreciate your accomplishments along the road, no matter how tiny. This positive reinforcement strengthens your dedication to your flexibility objectives and raises morale.

Women over 50 who follow these rules for realistic goal setting can effectively increase their flexibility and get the myriad advantages of a limber body and greater range of motion. Remember, the path to increased flexibility is a marathon, not a sprint, so patience and perseverance are essential.

Overcoming Exercise Misconceptions

Flexibility exercises are frequently disregarded or misunderstood among women over the age of 50. There are some prevalent misunderstandings regarding flexibility training that might impede growth and keep people from reaching their fitness objectives.

Let's look at these common misunderstandings and how to overcome them in order to create a thorough flexibility training regimen designed exclusively for ladies over 50.

Flexibility Is Only for the Young: Many people feel that flexibility training is only beneficial for young athletes or dancers. However, preserving flexibility becomes increasingly important as we age. It promotes joint mobility, lowers the chance of injury, and improves total functional movement, all of which are essential for preserving independence and quality of life.

Flexibility Workouts are time-consuming. Some may believe that flexibility training requires a substantial time commitment.

However, even brief, frequent stretching sessions can result in substantial flexibility gains over time. Flexibility exercises, such as stretching while watching TV or before bedtime, might help make it easier and more pleasurable.

Flexibility Training is Boring: Many people find standard static stretching regimens tedious and uninteresting. However, there are some entertaining and dynamic flexibility exercises that may be included in a training routine.

Yoga, Pilates, tai chi, and dancing all enhance flexibility while also providing mental relaxation and stress reduction.

Flexibility workouts are only for flexible people. Contrary to common opinion, flexibility training is not only for people who are naturally flexible. Stretching exercises may help everybody, regardless of flexibility level. With persistent practice, people can progressively enhance their range of motion and flexibility.

To combat these preconceptions, women over 50 should incorporate flexibility activities in their fitness regimen. This can involve a variety of static and dynamic stretches, yoga postures, and mobility exercises suited to their unique requirements and skills.

Women over 50 can improve their physical health, lower their risk of injury, and increase their quality of life by including

flexibility training into their total exercise
regimen.

Chapter 2: Assessing and Creating an Exercise Environment

Creating a fitness environment designed specifically for women over 50, with a focus on flexibility movements, necessitates thorough assessment and strategic planning.

Flexibility is essential for preserving mobility, avoiding accidents, and improving general well-being in this population. Here's a thorough strategy for assessing and creating an exercise setting suited to flexibility training for women over 50.

Assessment of requirements: Begin by learning about the target demographic's unique requirements and limits. Conduct surveys, interviews, and consultations to learn about their fitness objectives, current health concerns, and any past injuries.

Accessibility and Safety: Make sure the workout area is easily accessible and safe for ladies over 50. To avoid accidents or falls, provide handrails, nonslip flooring, appropriate lighting, and clear walkways.

Flexibility training equipment includes yoga mats, resistance bands, foam rollers, and stability balls. Include equipment that caters to all fitness levels and capabilities.

Create a warm and comfortable setting that fosters involvement while reducing anxiety. Consider temperature control, ventilation, and ambient music to help you relax and focus throughout your exercises.

Qualified Instructors: Ensure that instructors have experience dealing with older persons and are familiar with adjusting activities for different fitness levels and health issues. Encourage continual professional development to keep current with best practices.

organized Programs: Create organized flexibility programs exclusively for women over 50. Include a variety of stretching exercises for main muscle groups, joint mobility drills, and relaxation strategies such as deep breathing or meditation.

Progressive Overload: Gradually increase the intensity and complexity of flexibility exercises to challenge participants while avoiding injury. To increase efficacy while minimizing strain, emphasize appropriate technique and alignment.

Community Support: Organizing group courses, social gatherings, or online forums can help participants feel more connected and supported. Encourage social contact and reciprocal support to boost motivation and commitment to the program.

Regular Evaluation: Continuously monitor and assess the success of the exercise environment and programs based on participant input, performance metrics, and health outcomes. Make changes as needed to improve performance and satisfaction.

By adhering to these criteria, you may establish an exercise environment that enables women over 50 to increase flexibility, mobility, and general health, therefore improving their quality of life and fostering long-term well-being.

Evaluating Fitness Level and Health

Evaluating fitness levels and staying healthy are critical components of total well-being, especially for women over 50. Flexibility activities are essential for improving mobility, reducing injuries, and maintaining general physical health in this group.

To begin, determining one's degree of fitness requires an assessment of flexibility. Simple exams like the sit-and-reach test or shoulder flexibility evaluations can give information about one's current flexibility level. Regular assessments enable individuals to monitor their development and identify areas for improvement.

Flexibility workouts for women over 50 should include stretching, yoga, and mobility exercises. These exercises serve to reduce stiffness, improve joint range of motion, and increase overall flexibility. Dynamic stretches before a workout and static stretches afterward can significantly increase flexibility while lowering the chance of injury.

Yoga, which focuses on controlled movements and deep stretches, is especially useful for women over 50. It not only increases flexibility but also improves balance, core strength, and mental health. Regular yoga practice can help you gain more flexibility and awareness of your body.

Mobility exercises such as hip circles, shoulder rolls, and ankle rotations are essential for joint health and function. These exercises target particular parts of the body that are prone to stiffness and tightness, increasing total flexibility and lowering the chance of injury.

Furthermore, Flexibility training must be tailored to each individual's specific demands and skills. Women over 50 may have various degrees of flexibility and mobility, therefore workouts should be tailored accordingly. Gradually increasing the intensity and duration of workouts guarantees consistent growth without overtraining.

Women over 50 should evaluate their fitness levels and prioritize flexibility training to maintain optimal health.

Women who incorporate a range of stretching, yoga, and mobility exercises into their routine can increase their flexibility, minimize their risk of injury, and improve their general well-being. Regular assessments and modifications guarantee that fitness objectives are met safely and efficiently.

Safe Home Exercise Setup

Creating a safe home exercise setting for women over 50, with an emphasis on flexibility training, is critical for maintaining general health and avoiding injury. Here's a full guide to creating a safe and successful exercise environment:

Choose the Right Space: To workout, find a well-lit, large location with a level surface. Avoid clutter and make sure there is adequate space to walk around easily.

Invest in Proper Equipment: While flexibility exercises may not require much equipment, having a few crucial items will help you get most out of your workouts.

Consider purchasing a yoga mat for cushioning and stability, resistance bands for extra resistance, and yoga blocks for support during stretching.

Ensure appropriate lighting and ventilation. Choose a room that receives natural light or install bright, adjustable lighting. Also, provide appropriate ventilation to avoid overheating and discomfort during workouts.

Remain Hydrated: Keep a water bottle nearby to remain hydrated during your workout. Proper hydration is critical, especially for women over 50, to retain energy and avoid dehydration.

Warm-Up and Cool-Down: Start each session with a mild warm-up to prepare your muscles and joints for activity. This might involve light aerobic exercises such as walking or marching in place, followed by dynamic stretches.

Similarly, after your workout, take a cool-down session to gradually drop your heart rate and stretch out your muscles.

Focus on Form and Technique: To avoid injury, keep your form and technique in check during workouts. Begin with easy motions and develop as your flexibility improves. If you're unsure, contact with a fitness specialist for advice.

Listen to Your Body: It is critical to listen to your body and respect its boundaries. If you feel any pain or discomfort during a workout, stop immediately and check your technique. Pushing through discomfort can cause harm, so always emphasize safety.

Modify as Needed: Don't be afraid to change workouts to meet your own requirements and talents. Use supports such as chairs or walls to help you balance, and select exercises that are both comfortable and effective for you.

Women over 50 can benefit from flexibility training while reducing their risk of injury by following these instructions and creating a safe home exercise environment. Remember to emphasize safety, listen to your body, and stick to your workout regimen for best results.

Mindfulness Integration

Mindfulness integration in flexibility workouts for women over 50 is a comprehensive strategy to improving physical and mental well-being.

It combines mindful activities and flexibility exercises to increase awareness, reduce stress, and promote general health. Here's a detailed explanation of how mindfulness might be included in flexibility training for this demographic:

Breath Awareness: Start each flexibility workout by concentrating on your breath. Encourage women to focus on their breath, breathing deeply through the nose and expelling gently through the mouth.

This helps to focus the mind, boost oxygen flow, and promote relaxation.

Body Scan: Use a body scan technique to improve bodily awareness. Encourage people to pay attention to each part of their body, from head to toe, and note any areas of tension or discomfort.

Encourage them to release tension with each exhale, resulting in a sensation of relaxation and openness throughout the body.

Mindful Movement: Guide participants through flexibility exercises while stressing the relationship between movement and breath.

Encourage slow, deliberate motions, concentrating on the feelings in the body as you stretch and release. This promotes present-moment awareness and strengthens the mind-body connection.

Acceptance and nonjudgment: Develop a nonjudgmental attitude toward the body's limits and capabilities. Encourage women to approach flexibility exercises with compassion and care for themselves, letting go of any expectations or self-criticism. This fosters a sense of inner serenity and self-compassion.

Gratitude Practice: Incorporate a gratitude practice into your flexibility exercise program. Encourage participants to consider the parts of their bodies for which they are thankful, with a focus on strength, flexibility, and resilience. Cultivating appreciation boosts good feelings and promotes satisfaction.

Mindful Rest: After each flexibility workout, allow for some mindful rest or relaxation. Guide participants through a body scan or progressive muscle relaxation, allowing them to fully relax and absorb the benefits of their practice.

By including mindfulness into flexibility workouts for women over 50, we not only improve physical health but also foster mental and emotional well-being, allowing participants to age gracefully with energy and resilience.

Chapter 3: Daily Flexibility Exercises for Weight Loss

Maintaining flexibility is critical for general health and weight loss, particularly in women over 50.

Incorporating regular flexibility exercises into your program can improve mobility, minimize injury risk, and aid in weight reduction. Here's a complete guide to daily flexibility exercises designed for ladies over 50:

Stretching: Begin your day with a series of mild stretches that target key muscle groups. Concentrate on tight muscles in the hips, hamstrings, shoulders, and lower back. Hold each stretch for 15–30 seconds without jumping to prevent tension.

Yoga: Enjoy the advantages of yoga for flexibility and weight loss. Beginner-friendly positions include downward-facing dog, cat-cow stretch, and sitting forward bend. Yoga not only increases flexibility, but it also encourages relaxation and stress reduction.

Pilates: Incorporate Pilates into your regimen to strengthen your core muscles and increase flexibility. Pilates movements like as the hundred, roll-up, and spine twist promote stability and balance while improving range of motion.

Tai Chi: Learn the gentle motions of Tai Chi, which are believed to improve flexibility, balance, and mental health.

This ancient practice blends slow, flowing motions with deep breathing methods, making it excellent for women over 50 who want to enhance their flexibility and lose weight.

Foam rolling: Use a foam roller to relieve muscular tension and increase flexibility.

Roll softly over tight regions, using mild pressure to release knots and promote blood flow. Foam rolling can aid in recovery after exercise and reduce muscular tightness.

Dynamic Stretching: Include dynamic stretching in your warm-up regimen before exercising. Leg swings, arm circles, and torso twists can help increase blood flow to muscles and improve flexibility.

Regular Mobility Work: Incorporate mobility exercises into your everyday routine to keep your joints healthy and flexible. Activities such as shoulder circles, ankle rolls, and neck rotations serve to avoid stiffness and improve range of motion.

Women over 50 who incorporate these regular flexibility exercises into their regimen can help them lose weight while also improving their general health and mobility. Remember to listen to your body, start carefully, and gradually increase the intensity to minimize injury and optimize benefits.

Dynamic Warm-Up Routines

Dynamic warm-up practices are vital for women over 50, especially when it comes to flexibility training. These activities not only get the body ready for physical activity, but they also lower the chance of injury and increase overall performance.

Here is a thorough guide to active warm-up exercises created exclusively for women over 50, with a focus on flexibility.

Begin with mild rotations of the neck, shoulders, elbows, wrists, spine, hips, knees, and ankles. These exercises promote blood flow to the joints, improve mobility, and relieve stiffness.

Dynamic Stretching: Use dynamic stretches to simulate the motions you'll be doing during your workout. Stretches that target key muscular groups such as the hamstrings, quadriceps, calves, chest, back, and shoulders are ideal for increasing flexibility. Examples include leg swings, arm circles, hip circles, and trunk rotations.

Include exercises that require balance and stability, such as single-leg stands, heel-to-toe walks, and side-leg lifts. These exercises not only enhance proprioception but also assist in reducing falls, which are becoming increasingly prevalent as we age.

Cardiovascular Activation: Use mild cardiovascular activities such as brisk walking, marching in place, or low-impact aerobic motions to boost heart rate and blood supply to the muscles. This prepares the cardiovascular system for more vigorous action while increasing overall energy levels.

Incorporate Proprioceptive Drills: The body's knowledge of its location in space, known as proprioception, tends to deteriorate with age. Include movements like toe taps, ankle circles, and standing knee lifts to improve proprioception and lower the chance of falls and injuries.

Gradual Progression: Begin with gentler exercises, gradually increasing the intensity and range of motion as your body warms up. Listen to your body and avoid pushing through discomfort or suffering.

Mindful Breathing: During the warm-up, concentrate on deep, diaphragmatic breathing to oxygenate the muscles and relax the mind. This also helps to boost attention and concentration during exercise.

Women over 50 who incorporate these dynamic warm-up routines into their flexibility workouts may improve their performance, minimize their risk of injury, and reap the advantages of increased mobility and general well-being.

Always contact a healthcare expert before beginning any new workout regimen, especially if you have any underlying health concerns.

Targeted Stretching Techniques

As women age, maintaining flexibility becomes more crucial for their general health and well-being. Targeted stretching exercises can be especially useful for women over 50, since they help combat the natural loss of flexibility and mobility that comes with age.

Here's a whole guide on excellent stretching exercises designed exclusively for this demographic:

Start your flexibility training with a vigorous warm-up to boost blood flow to your muscles and prepare them for stretching. This can involve arm circles, leg swings, and slow running in place.

Joint Mobilization: Use mild joint mobilization exercises to increase joint mobility and decrease stiffness. This might include circular motions of the wrists, ankles, shoulders, and hips to lubricate the joints and improve range of motion.

Static Stretching: Use static stretching exercises to target key muscular areas such the hamstrings, quadriceps, calves, chest, shoulder, and back. To progressively build flexibility, hold each stretch for 20-30 seconds while breathing deeply and relaxing into it.

Foam rolling is a technique for releasing tension and stiffness in muscles via self-myofascial release. Roll carefully over tight places, pausing at any delicate points for deeper relief.

Yoga and Pilates: Add yoga and Pilates poses and movements to your flexibility regimen to increase balance, stability, and flexibility. Poses like downward dog, warrior II, and sitting spinal twist can help stretch and strengthen the body while also encouraging relaxation and stress reduction.

Prop-Assisted Stretching: Use props such as yoga blocks, straps, or stability balls to help you stretch and increase the intensity of the stretches.

This allows women over 50 to comfortably stretch deeper and enhance their flexibility without hurting or overexerting themselves.

Cool Down: After your flexibility training, gently cool down to assist relax the muscles and avoid stiffness. Slow, controlled movements and deep breathing might help you relax and recuperate.

Women over 50 who include these focused stretching exercises into their training program can increase flexibility, mobility, and general physical function and vitality for many years.

Low-Impact Cardiovascular Activities

Women over 50 should engage in low-impact cardiovascular activities to preserve heart health, improve circulation, and manage their weight.

These exercises are easy on the joints, making them suitable for anyone with joint problems or arthritis. Including flexibility activities in their program improves mobility, prevents injury, and promotes general health.

Low-Impact Cardiovascular Activities:

Walking: Walking is a simple yet efficient approach to get the heart rate up without putting too much strain on the joints. Women over 50 might begin with short walks and progressively increase the length and intensity.

Swimming: Swimming is an excellent low-impact workout that works the entire body. It promotes cardiovascular health, strengthens muscles, and increases flexibility. Water has inherent resistance, making it ideal for ladies with arthritis or joint discomfort.

Riding: Whether done outdoors or on a stationary bike, riding is easy on the joints and provides a terrific cardiovascular exercise. It strengthens the legs, increases endurance, and is readily adjustable to suit different fitness levels.

Elliptical Training: The elliptical machine is a low-impact alternative to running and jogging. It provides a full-body workout, focusing on the arms, legs, and core muscles.

Adjusting the resistance level enables for personalized workouts based on fitness objectives and skills.

Flexible Workouts

Yoga is good for women over 50 since it increases flexibility, balance, and strength. Gentle yoga positions serve to relieve muscular and joint stiffness, promote relaxation, and reduce stress.

Pilates emphasizes core strength, flexibility, and body awareness. It uses regulated movements and breathing methods to enhance posture, mobility, and stability.

Tai Chi is a benign martial art based on slow, flowing motions and deep breathing. It improves balance, coordination, and flexibility while also relaxing and lowering anxiety.

Stretching: Including regular stretching exercises in your workout program helps you retain flexibility and avoid muscular stiffness. The neck, shoulders, back, hips, and legs are all prime targets.

Low-impact cardiovascular activity and flexibility training are critical for women over 50 to preserve general health and well-being. By implementing these activities into their daily routine, people can enhance their heart health, mobility, and quality of life.

Chapter 4: Core Strength for Stability and Posture

Core strength is essential for stability and posture, especially for women over 50 looking to preserve flexibility and general health. A strong core not only supports the spine, but it also improves balance, lowers the chance of injury, and promotes functional mobility.

The importance of core strength:

Stability: A strong core offers a solid foundation for all motions, whether you're bending down to pick up something or reaching aloft.

This stability is critical for maintaining balance, especially as we age and our equilibrium begins to deteriorate.

Posture: The core muscles support the spine and keep it in appropriate alignment, minimizing slouching and lowering the risk of back discomfort. Good posture not only looks great, but it also improves breathing and circulation.

Core Strengthening Exercises:
Planks: This traditional exercise works the whole core, including the abs, obliques, and lower back. Begin with brief holds and progressively increase them as your strength develops.

Russian Twists: Sit on the floor, knees bent, and spin your torso from side to side while gripping a weight or medicine ball. This exercise works the obliques and increases rotational stability.

Bird Dogs: Start in a hands-and-knees posture and extend one arm and the opposing leg at the same time, keeping your core engaged. This workout strengthens the entire core and improves balance and coordination.

Bridge: Lie on your back, knees bent and feet flat on the floor, then raise your hips off the ground while squeezing your glutes and working your core. This workout focuses on the lower back, glutes, and hamstrings.

Integrating core strengthening exercises with flexibility training is crucial for women over 50 to maintain a healthy fitness program.

A strong core promotes optimal alignment during stretches and prevents injury by supporting joints. improved posture from core strengthening can increase the efficiency of flexibility exercises, allowing for a wider range of motion and lowering the risk of strain.

Women over the age of 50 can improve their general health and well-being by focusing on core strength, posture, and flexibility exercises.

Pilates-inspired Core Workouts

As women get older, keeping flexibility and core strength becomes more crucial for their general health and vitality. Pilates-inspired core workouts are a great technique to address these regions, since they provide a holistic training strategy that improves flexibility, muscular strength, and posture.

Here's a thorough explanation of why Pilates-inspired core workouts are useful for women over 50:

1. Concentrate on Core Strength: Pilates movements emphasize the core muscles, which include the deep abdominal muscles, obliques, and lower back. Strengthening these muscles helps to stabilize the spine, enhance stability, and lowers the chance of injuries, particularly common ones like lower back discomfort.

2. **_Improves Flexibility:_** Pilates uses dynamic stretches and motions to increase flexibility throughout the body, particularly the spine, hips, and shoulders. Improved flexibility not only enhances range of motion, but also helps to preserve general mobility and avoid stiffness caused by age.

3. **_Low-Impact Exercise:_** Many Pilates movements are regulated and low-impact, making them excellent for women over 50 who may have joint problems or other mobility limitations. This mild approach to training minimizes the danger of strain or injury while yet offering a demanding workout.

4. _Improves Posture:_ As people age, they typically develop poor posture, which causes discomfort and agony. Pilates exercises emphasize alignment and good body mechanics, which assist to rectify postural abnormalities and produce a more upright, balanced stance.

5.   *Mind-Body   Connection:*   Pilates promotes a thoughtful approach to movement, stressing focus, breath control, and physical awareness. This mind-body link not only improves workout efficacy, but it also promotes relaxation and mental health.

Incorporating Pilates-inspired core movements into a regular fitness regimen can provide considerable advantages for women over 50, including increased flexibility, strength, and vitality.

Pilates, whether performed in a group class, under the supervision of a qualified teacher, or at home using online resources, is a safe and effective approach to promote healthy aging and maintain an active lifestyle.

Yoga Poses for Core Stability

Maintaining core stability and flexibility is especially important as we age. Yoga is a gentle yet effective technique to attain these aims, tailored particularly to the requirements of women over 50. Here are some thorough yoga poses designed to improve core stability and flexibility in this demographic:

Plank Pose (Phalakasana): Start in a push-up posture, putting your wrists beneath your shoulders. Engage your core and keep your body in a straight line from head to heels. Hold for 30 seconds to a minute, progressively increasing as your strength grows.

This position works the whole core, including the abdominals, back, and shoulders, and improves posture.

Bridge Pose (Setu Bandhasana): Lie on your back, knees bent, feet hip-width apart.

With your feet and arm pressing on the mat,your hips should be lifted towards the ceiling. Maintain parallel thighs while engaging your glutes and core. Hold for 30 seconds to a minute before releasing softly. Bridge position strengthens the core, back, and glutes while increasing spinal flexibility.

Cat-Cow Stretch (Marjaryasana-Bitilasana): Begin on your hands and knees, wrists under shoulders, knees under hips. Inhale, arching your back and raising your tailbone and head to the ceiling (cow position).

Exhale while curving your spine towards the sky and burying your chin into your chest (cat stance). Flow through these positions for 5-10 breaths. Cat-cow stretch increases spine flexibility and core stability.

Seated Twist (Ardha Matsyendrasana): Sit upright with your legs outstretched. Bend your right knee and position the foot outside the left thigh.

Inhale, stretch the spine, and then exhale while rotating to the right, placing your left elbow outside the right knee. Hold for 30 seconds and then switch sides. Seated twists promote spinal mobility, which improves core stability and digestion.

Downward-Facing Dog (Adho Mukha Svanasana): Beggin on your hands and knees, then elevate your hips to the ceiling while straightening your arms and legs into an inverted V shape.

Press your heels to the floor while engaging your core and stretching your spine. Hold for 30 seconds to a minute, focusing on deep breathing. The downward dog exercise stretches the spine, hamstrings, and shoulders while strengthening the core and arms.

Incorporating these yoga positions into a daily practice can help women over 50 improve their core stability and flexibility, supporting overall health and effective mobility. Remember to listen to your body and adjust positions as needed for safety and comfort.

Functional Training for Balance

Functional balance training is vital, especially for women over 50, because it helps them retain stability, mobility, and independence in their everyday activities. Incorporating flexibility exercises into functional training improves general balance and lowers the chance of falling or injury.

Flexibility exercises for women over 50 should aim to improve joint mobility and muscle suppleness. Dynamic stretches, such as leg swings and arm circles, serve to enhance range of motion and prepare the body to move. Static stretches, such as hamstring and calf stretches, are useful for extending muscles and increasing flexibility.

Yoga and Pilates are good flexibility workouts for women over 50 because they combine strength and flexibility. Yoga positions including downward dog, warrior II, and tree pose help you enhance your balance, flexibility, and core strength. Pilates movements like the hundred, spine stretch forward, and single leg circles work particular muscle groups while increasing flexibility and stability.

Including balancing exercises in functional training improves general stability and coordination. Balance activities including single-leg stands, heel-to-toe walks, and stability ball exercises test proprioception and improve stabilizing muscles. These workouts may be tailored to specific fitness levels and skills.

Incorporating resistance training into functional workouts also increases muscular strength, which is essential for maintaining balance and stability. Squats, lunges, and calf raises work important muscle groups while boosting bone density and joint health.

When it comes to functional balance and flexibility training, consistency is essential.

Try to include these exercises into your program at least 2-3 times each week, progressively increasing the intensity and complexity as your strength and balance improve.

Remember to listen to your body and speak with a healthcare expert before beginning any new fitness regimen, especially if you have any pre-existing health issues or injuries.

Women over 50 who prioritize functional exercise for balance and flexibility can improve their overall quality of life and retain their independence as they get older.

Chapter 5: Enhancing Balance and Coordination

Improving balance and coordination is critical for general well-being, particularly among women over 50.

Our bodies typically degrade in these areas as we age, but tailored flexibility training may greatly improve balance and coordination, increasing quality of life and lowering the risk of falls and accidents.

Yoga: Yoga is an excellent approach to increasing flexibility, balance, and coordination. Tree Pose, Warrior Pose, and Downward Dog stretch muscles while also challenging balance and coordination. Regular practice can improve stability and body awareness.

Pilates emphasizes core strength, which is necessary for balance and stability. Pilates movements frequently involve exact control and coordination, which aids with general body awareness and alignment.

Stretching: Including stretching exercises in your program helps increase flexibility and range of motion, which can help with balance and coordination. Concentrate on stretches that target key muscular groups, such as the hamstrings, quadriceps, calves, and shoulders.

Simple balancing exercises, such as standing on one leg, heel-to-toe walking, or utilizing a balance board, can assist strengthen stabilizing muscles and increase coordination. Begin with basic exercises and progressively increase in difficulty as your balance improves.

Functional training involves mimicking ordinary motions in exercises to develop functional balance and coordination. Squats, lunges, and step-ups are examples of exercises that need both stability and strength.

Consistency and Progress: Practicing flexibility exercises on a regular basis is essential for improving balance and coordination. Start softly and progressively increase the intensity and difficulty over time to keep the body challenged and progressing.

Women over 50 who incorporate these focused flexibility workouts into their routine can improve their balance and coordination, resulting in greater overall health and a lower chance of falls and accidents.

Regular practice, along with good technique and development, can help individuals maintain independence and vigor as they age.

Thorough Mobility Training

Mobility exercise is essential for women over 50 to retain flexibility, avoid accidents, and enhance their general quality of life. This holistic workout method focuses on improving range of motion, joint health, and functional movement patterns.

Here's a complete overview of comprehensive mobility training, particularly geared to ladies over 50:

Warm-up: Start with an active warm-up that increases blood flow and prepares the body for exercise. To release muscles and joints, use exercises such as arm circles, leg swings, and hip rotations.

Mobility exercises that target particular joints can help develop flexibility and reduce stiffness. To increase overall mobility, use exercises such as neck circles, shoulder rolls, wrist rotations, spine twists, hip circles, knee circles, and ankle circles.

Flexibility Workouts: Combine static and dynamic stretching workouts to increase flexibility. Concentrate on large muscular groups such as the hamstrings, quadriceps, calves, chest, shoulders, and back.

Hold each stretch for 20–30 seconds, then alternate between static and dynamic stretches to increase flexibility and range of motion.

Balance and Stability Training: Use balance exercises to increase stability and lessen the chance of falling.

Include activities like single-leg stands, heel-to-toe walks, and balance board exercises to test your proprioception and enhance your general balance.

Functional Movement Patterns: Focus on functional motions that are similar to everyday tasks. Squats, lunges, hinges, pushes, pulls, and twists are all workouts that can help you increase your mobility and strength in real life.

Progressive Overload: Gradually increase the intensity and complexity of mobility exercises to keep the body challenged and adaptable. To make development over time, incorporate changes, increased resistance, or longer periods.

Cool Down and Recovery: End the exercise with a cooldown to reduce heart rate and enhance recovery. Gentle stretching and foam rolling can help relieve muscular tension and promote relaxation.

Women over 50 who incorporate extensive mobility training into their workout program can increase flexibility, lower the chance of injury, and improve general well-being.

Consistency and good technique are essential for optimizing the advantages of mobility exercise on long-term health and energy.

Tai Chi for Balance

Tai Chi, an ancient Chinese martial art, has various benefits for women over 50, notably in terms of balance and flexibility.

As women age, keeping balance becomes increasingly important to avoid falls and accidents, and Tai Chi offers an excellent answer.

To begin, Tai Chi emphasizes slow, controlled motions that recruit several muscle groups, therefore increasing flexibility.

The soft, flowing motions stretch the body, increasing joint mobility and range of motion, which is especially good for ladies suffering from age-related stiffness.

Tai Chi improves proprioception, or the body's sense of its location in space. This increased awareness allows women over 50 to retain greater balance and coordination, lowering their chance of falling.

Tai Chi teaches them how to appropriately distribute their weight and change their posture, which leads to increased stability in everyday tasks.

Tai Chi utilizes breathing methods to promote relaxation and stress reduction. Women over 50 are more likely to experience stress and anxiety, so these breathing exercises can generate a sense of peace and well-being, improving overall mental and physical health.

Tai Chi also develops mindfulness, which helps the mind focus on the present moment and improve attention.

This mental element is critical for women over 50 since it keeps them intellectually alert and attentive to their surroundings, lowering the risk of accidents caused by distraction or lack of attention.

Tai Chi is a wonderful alternative for ladies over 50 who want to enhance their balance and flexibility. Its gentle, low-impact motions are a safe and effective approach to build muscle, increase flexibility, and promote general health.

Women who incorporate Tai Chi into their training program might experience improved balance, less stress, and more confidence in their everyday activities.

Proprioceptive Exercises

As women age, maintaining flexibility becomes increasingly important for their general health and mobility.

Proprioceptive exercises are important for increasing flexibility and stability, which promote independence and reduce the chance of injury.

These workouts aim to improve proprioception, which is the body's capacity to perceive its location in space. Here's a whole guide on proprioceptive exercises designed for ladies over 50:

Balance Board Exercises: Using a balance board tests proprioception by forcing the body to steady itself. Simple exercises like standing on one leg or doing mild motions on the board will help you improve your balance and stability.

Pilates emphasizes core strength, alignment, and control. Many Pilates exercises involve precise motions that need knowledge of body posture, which helps to improve proprioception while simultaneously increasing flexibility.

Resistance Band exercises: Adding resistance bands to exercises creates an element of instability, encouraging the body to utilize stabilizing muscles. Exercises such as lateral leg lifts and arm curls with bands not only increase strength but also enhance proprioception.

Stability Ball Exercises: Performing exercises on a stability ball necessitates regular modifications to maintain equilibrium. Simple ball exercises, such as sitting leg lifts or bridges, activate core muscles and increase proprioception.

Dynamic stretching entails going through a full range of motion under controlled conditions. Arm circles, leg swings, and torso twists increase flexibility while engaging proprioceptive receptors.

Mindful Movement Practices: Mindfulness-based exercises such as Feldenkrais or Alexander Technique emphasize body awareness and effective movement patterns. These techniques can help women over 50 have a better knowledge of their bodies and increase proprioception.

Incorporating proprioceptive exercises into a regular workout program can improve flexibility, balance, and general well-being in women over 50. These workouts promote good aging and activity by pushing the body's proprioceptive system.

Balance Challenges in Daily Life

Achieving balance in daily life is a complicated endeavor that includes physical, mental, and emotional stability. Maintaining balance becomes even more important for women over 50 as their bodies age and lifestyle demands shift.

Flexibility is a critical component of physical balance, as it helps to improve mobility, reduce injuries, and promote general well-being.

Flexibility training designed for women over 50 is vital for meeting the unique demands of aging bodies. These workouts aim to improve joint mobility, increase range of motion, and reduce stiffness.

Combining workouts that target multiple muscle groups and movement patterns can help women over 50 maintain or increase their flexibility.

Yoga stands out as a fantastic option for improving flexibility in women over 50. Its soft yet efficient poses not only increase flexibility, but also strength and balance. Yoga also promotes mental relaxation and stress alleviation, which improves general well-being.

Pilates is another good alternative, as it emphasizes core strength, stability, and flexibility through regulated movements. Its low-impact nature makes it appropriate for people of all fitness levels, including those who have joint problems or injuries.

including stretching exercises into regular activities will help you retain flexibility. Simple stretches, such as toe touches, shoulder rolls, and side stretches, can help relieve tension and increase flexibility in important regions including the hamstrings, shoulders, and spine.

Women over 50 should tackle flexibility training with care and regularity. Progress may be sluggish, but with focus and patience, significant gains can be made over time.

Consulting with a fitness expert or physical therapist may also give specific coaching while ensuring that activities are safe and effective.

Women over 50 who face balance issues in their everyday lives must prioritize physical health, especially flexibility.

Women may improve their mobility, lower their risk of injury, and have a better quality of life as they age by adding specialized flexibility workouts such as yoga, Pilates, and regular stretching regimens.

Chapter 6: Joint Health and Flexibility

Maintaining joint health and flexibility is critical for general wellness, especially as we age. Prioritizing flexibility training can help women over 50 reduce stiffness, lower their risk of injury, and improve their mobility in everyday activities.

A well-balanced exercise plan that combines stretching, weight training, and low-impact aerobic workouts is critical for improving joint health and flexibility.

Stretching exercises aim to increase range of motion in joints and muscles, promote flexibility, and reduce stiffness.

Arm circles, leg swings, and torso twists are great for warming up the muscles and preparing them for more strenuous exercise.

Yoga and Pilates are also quite useful for women over 50 since they emphasize both flexibility and strength. These techniques stress controlled motions and precise alignment, which can help prevent injuries and improve general posture.

Yoga also includes breathing methods that promote relaxation and reduce tension, which are good to general joint health.

Strength training routines, such as bodyweight exercises, resistance band workouts, and light dumbbell exercises, are critical for maintaining muscle mass and joint function.

Strong muscles serve to support and protect the joints from harm. Concentrate on workouts that work key muscular groups such the legs, arms, back, and core.

Low-impact cardio workouts, such as walking, swimming, or cycling, are excellent for boosting cardiovascular health without placing undue strain on joints. These activities enhance blood flow to the muscles and joints, which promotes healing and decreases inflammation.

Women over 50 can benefit significantly from including flexibility activities into their regular fitness plan. To avoid overexertion and injury, exercises should be started initially and progressively increased in intensity and length.

Consulting with a healthcare expert or a trained fitness instructor can help you create a training plan that is tailored to your specific requirements and limits.

Joint health and flexibility are critical components of total wellbeing, especially in women over 50. Women who incorporate stretching, weight training, and low-impact aerobic workouts into their daily routines can increase joint mobility, reduce stiffness, and improve their overall quality of life.

Joint-Specific Stretching

As women age, maintaining flexibility becomes more important for their general health and well-being. Joint-specific stretching is a focused strategy for increasing flexibility, mobility, and joint function that is customized to the specific requirements of women over 50.

This thorough approach focuses on stretching particular joints to increase range of motion and lower the chance of injury.

Why should you stretch your joints specifically?

Joint-specific stretching understands that each joint has a unique range of motion and flexibility requirements. As women age, their joints may stiffen owing to factors including decreasing synovial fluid production and changes in muscle suppleness.

This strategy increases flexibility development by focusing on specific joints such the hips, shoulders, and spine.

Benefits for Women Over 50:

For women over 50, joint-specific stretching gives several benefits.

Improved Mobility: Increased flexibility enables smoother, more fluid movements, making daily tasks easier and lowering the chance of falls and accidents.

Pain Relief: Targeted stretching can help relieve joint pain and stiffness, increasing overall joint health and comfort.

Stretching tight muscles around the spine and shoulders helps improve posture and relieve tension on the back and neck.

Injury Prevention: By strengthening flexibility in certain joints, women can lower their risk of strains, sprains, and other musculoskeletal injuries during exercise and daily activities.

Key Techniques

Prioritize stretching activities for joints that are tight or causing discomfort.

Hold and Breathe: Hold each stretch for 15-30 seconds, breathing deeply to promote relaxation and deepening the stretch.

Begin with easy stretches and gradually increase the intensity and length over time to avoid overstretching or injury.

Include a range of stretching exercises aimed at different joints and muscle groups to improve general flexibility and mobility.

Joint-specific stretching is an important part of flexibility workouts for women over 50, as it provides focused advantages that improve joint health, mobility, and general well-being. Women who include these practices into their daily exercise program can preserve flexibility, avoid injuries, and have an active and meaningful life as they age.

Foam Rolling for Joint Health

Foam rolling is a highly effective practice for improving joint health, especially in people over 50 who may have diminished flexibility and mobility owing to age-related changes in the body.

This self-myofascial release technique uses a foam roller to provide pressure to tight muscles and fascia, therefore improving circulation, reducing muscular tension, and increasing total joint mobility.

Flexibility exercises are essential for women over 50 who want to keep their joints healthy and avoid accidents.

Foam rolling may be added to their workout program to target particular areas of stiffness and discomfort, such as the hips, knees, and shoulders. Women can enhance their range of motion and relieve stiffness by foam rolling these regions on a regular basis, making daily tasks simpler and more pleasant.

Foam rolling helps to break down adhesions and knots in the muscles and fascia, which can limit movement and cause joint discomfort.

Women over 50 can benefit from increased flexibility and reduced stiffness in their joints by releasing these tight places, allowing them to move more easily and comfortably.

In addition to improving joint health, foam rolling can help with injury prevention and recovery.

Women over 50 who incorporate foam rolling into their flexibility workouts can lower their risk of strains, sprains, and other common problems caused by tight muscles and reduced mobility.

To maximize the benefits of foam rolling for joint health, women over 50 should add it into their normal exercise program, ideally before and after exercises.

 They should concentrate on specific areas of tightness and pain, rolling gently and methodically over each muscle group for 1-2 minutes.

Foam rolling is an effective method for improving joint health and flexibility in women over 50.

By adopting this method into their workout program, individuals may enhance their range of motion, reduce stiffness, and lower their risk of injury, allowing them to remain active and independent as they age.

Nutrition for Joint Support

A proper diet is critical for joint health, particularly for women over 50, who may face age-related changes and an increased risk of joint problems.

Incorporating particular nutrients into your diet can help preserve joint flexibility and lower your risk of joint-related disorders like osteoarthritis. Here's a detailed reference on the diet for joint support geared toward women over 50, as well as flexibility exercises:

Omega-3 Fatty Acids: Found in fatty fish such as salmon, flaxseeds, and walnuts, omega-3s have anti-inflammatory qualities that can help with joint pain and stiffness.

Antioxidants: Colorful fruits and vegetables, such as berries, oranges, and spinach, contain antioxidants like vitamin C and E, which fight oxidative stress and decrease joint inflammation.

Calcium and Vitamin D: Calcium-rich foods such as dairy products, fortified plant-based milk, and leafy greens, when paired with vitamin D from sunshine exposure and fortified foods, promote bone density and joint health.

Collagen: As we age, collagen synthesis decreases, affecting joint health. Consume collagen-rich foods such as bone broth, chicken skin, and fish skin, or try taking supplements to improve joint flexibility and suppleness.

Protein: Lean protein foods such as chicken, tofu, and lentils include amino acids that are necessary for the development and repair of joint tissues.

Hydration: Adequate water intake keeps joints lubricated and improves overall joint function.

Everyday,a minimum of at least eight glasses of water should be aimed at

In addition to healthy nutrition, women over 50 should engage in regular flexibility workouts to preserve joint mobility and prevent stiffness. Incorporate yoga, tai chi, and Pilates into your workout program, with an emphasis on mild stretches for the major muscle groups and joints.

These exercises increase flexibility, balance, and posture while decreasing the likelihood of falls and accidents.

Aim for at least 30 minutes of flexibility exercises on most days of the week, progressively increasing the intensity and length as tolerated. Consult a healthcare physician or a trained fitness instructor to create a personalized nutrition and exercise plan based on your unique needs and health state.

Chapter 7: Holistic Health Approaches

Holistic health stresses the interdependence of the mind, body, and spirit, fostering complete well-being rather than simply preventing sickness.

For women over 50, adding flexibility training to their general health regimen is critical for preserving mobility, reducing injuries, and improving quality of life.

Flexibility exercises aim to improve the range of motion in joints and muscles, which typically decreases with age. Here are thorough and detailed ways to flexibility training designed exclusively for ladies over 50:

Stretching Routines: Start with mild stretching exercises that target key muscle groups such the shoulders, back, hips, and legs. Combine static stretches (holding a position for 15-30 seconds) with dynamic stretches (moving through a range of motion). To enhance efficacy and limit the chance of damage, focus on deep breathing and relaxation throughout each stretch.

Yoga and Pilates use a comprehensive approach to flexibility and strength training, emphasizing controlled movements, good alignment, and breath awareness. Classes for elders or beginners sometimes stress adaptations and props to meet individual needs and abilities.

Tai Chi and Qigong are ancient Chinese practices that use gentle motions, meditation, and breathing to promote balance, flexibility, and mental clarity. Tai Chi and Qigong are especially good for older persons since they are low-impact and adaptable to all fitness levels.

Swimming, water aerobics, and aqua yoga are examples of aquatic workouts that provide a supportive environment for developing flexibility while reducing joint stress. The buoyancy of water decreases the danger of damage while still allowing for complete range of motion.

Mind-Body Connection: Use mindfulness practices like meditation, deep breathing exercises, or guided imagery to relax, reduce tension, and increase flexibility. Cultivating a strong mind-body connection can increase flexibility and well-being.

Women over 50 who incorporate these holistic flexibility workouts into their routine may improve their physical health, emotional well-being, and general quality of life, adopting holistic health concepts for healthy aging and vitality.

Mind-Body Practices

Mind-body activities include a wide range of strategies that combine mental and physical components to achieve overall health. These methods acknowledge the interdependence of the mind and body, stressing their powerful effect on one another.

Mind-body practices range from ancient traditions to current therapies, providing comprehensive approaches to improving health, managing stress, and cultivating inner peace.

1. *Meditation:* Meditation entails training the mind to focus and redirect thoughts, resulting in calm and increased awareness. Techniques range from mindfulness meditation, which promotes present-moment awareness, to transcendental meditation, which employs mantra repetition. According to research, meditation decreases stress, improves emotional management, and boosts cognitive performance.

2. *Yoga:* Developed in ancient India, yoga combines physical postures (asanas), breathing techniques (pranayama), and meditation to enhance both physical and mental well-being.

Regular practice increases flexibility, strength, and balance while lowering tension and anxiety. Hatha, Vinyasa, and Kundalini yoga styles are designed to meet a variety of requirements and interests.

3. *Biofeedback:* Biofeedback uses electronic sensors to track physiological processes including heart rate, muscular tension, and brain activity. Individuals learn to actively manage these functions via visual or auditory input, which reduces tension and promotes relaxation. Biofeedback techniques are utilized in therapeutic settings to treat a variety of disorders, including anxiety, chronic pain, and hypertension.

4. *Progressive Muscle calm (PMR):* PMR entails gradually tensing and releasing various muscle groups in order to relieve physical stress and produce calm. PMR increases anxiety, sleep quality, and general well-being by enhancing body awareness and relieving muscle tension.

Mind-body techniques provide comprehensive approaches to health and wellbeing by combining mental and physical components. Incorporating meditation, yoga, Tai Chi, biofeedback, or progressive muscle relaxation techniques into daily life can result in increased harmony, resilience, and energy.

Rest and Recovery

Rest and recuperation are critical components of any effective training or exercise program. They play an important function in helping the body adapt and progress, whether you're a top athlete or a casual gym user.

Understanding the value of rest and recuperation may help you perform better, avoid injuries, and improve your general health.

Rest refers to the period of time when you are not actively participating in physical activities. It is critical to enable the body to recover and restore itself after exercise.

This includes getting enough sleep every night, because sleep is when the body performs vital functions like muscle repair, hormone control, and memory consolidation.

Recovery, on the other hand, refers to particular procedures and practices designed to improve the body's ability to recover from exercise-induced stress.

This may involve foam rolling, stretching, massage, and contrast water treatment. These approaches enhance circulation, reduce muscular tension, and alleviate discomfort, allowing for speedier recovery.

One of the key advantages of rest and recuperation is the avoidance of overtraining. Pushing the body too hard without getting enough rest can lead to poor performance, increased injury risk, and burnout.

By including regular rest days into your training routine and prioritizing recovery activities, you can maintain a balanced approach to fitness and prevent overtaxing your body.

Relaxation and recuperation are required for peak performance. Giving your body time to rest helps it to adapt to the stress of exercise, resulting in increased strength, endurance, and general fitness. Without adequate recuperation, you may not get the expected benefits from your exercise efforts.

Rest and recuperation are essential components of any training regimen. By adopting proper rest intervals and efficient recovery procedures, you may improve your performance, avoid injuries, and promote long-term health and well-being.

Prioritizing rest and recuperation is not a sign of weakness, but rather a sound strategy for attaining your fitness objectives safely and successfully.

Maintaining Motivation

Maintaining motivation is essential for attaining long-term objectives and staying on target. Whether you're seeking personal improvement, career achievement, or physical objectives, here are some complete tactics for staying motivated:

Define concise, attainable goals with clear dates. Break them down into smaller, more achievable tasks so you can readily track your progress.

Find Your Why: Understand the motivations behind your aspirations. Connecting emotionally to the result boosts intrinsic drive and perseverance in difficult situations.

Celebrate Small Wins: Recognize and celebrate each milestone achieved along the road. Small triumphs offer a sense of achievement and motivate further improvement.

Create a Support System: Surround yourself with friends, family, or mentors who will encourage and motivate you. Share your goals with them to ensure responsibility and encouragement.

Maintain a positive perspective by concentrating on success, learning from setbacks, and engaging in self-compassion. Positive thinking increases resilience and keeps motivation high.

Visualize Success: Using visualization methods, vividly see yourself attaining your goals. Visualizing accomplishment boosts motivation and helps you overcome hurdles.

Establish pattern: Create a regular daily pattern that prioritizes things that are relevant to your goals. Habitual activities help to prevent decision fatigue and sustain momentum.

Seek inspiration: Read books, watch videos, or listen to podcasts on your hobbies or objectives. Learning about other people's experiences and success stories helps rekindle motivation.

Stay flexible: Be willing to adjust your strategy or aims as circumstances change. Flexibility enables continuous growth despite problems or unanticipated barriers.

Self-Care: Prioritize rest, diet, exercise, and leisure activities to preserve overall health. Physical and mental health have a direct influence on motivation.

Track Progress: Keep a notebook or utilize applications to track your progress on a regular basis. Seeing actual outcomes boosts motivation and gives useful feedback for development.

Reward Yourself: Create incentives for achieving key goals. Rewards give positive reinforcement and encourage ongoing effort.

Individuals who continuously apply these tactics may maintain motivation over time, overcome challenges, and achieve their most ambitious goals.

CONCLUSION

Flexibility workouts for women over 50 have several benefits that improve general health and well-being. As women age, keeping flexibility becomes increasingly crucial for preserving mobility, preventing accidents, and improving quality of life.

Stretching, yoga, and Pilates activities can help women increase their range of motion, relieve stiffness, and lower their risk of age-related illnesses like arthritis and osteoporosis.

Flexibility exercises improve posture and balance, which are critical for minimizing falls and preserving independence as women age.

Women may combat the consequences of sedentary lives and the reduction in flexibility that commonly comes with aging by integrating modest stretching and mobility exercises into their regimen. These workouts also assist to relieve joint pain and stiffness, allowing women to do their regular chores more easily and comfortably.

Flexibility exercises also improve mental health by lowering stress, encouraging relaxation, and increasing awareness. The mind-body connection developed via disciplines such as yoga and Pilates can enhance mood, raise self-confidence, and increase general resistance to age-related issues.

Flexibility training allow women to reconnect with their bodies, increase self-awareness, and feel empowered as they age.

Flexibility activities should be incorporated within a comprehensive fitness plan for women over 50 to promote lifespan and vitality. These exercises supplement aerobic and strength training regimens, resulting in a well-rounded approach to physical fitness that addresses the specific demands of aging bodies.

 By valuing flexibility, women may keep their independence, live an active lifestyle, and follow their hobbies far into their senior years.

Flexibility training have various benefits to women over 50, including better mobility, mental well-being, and general quality of life.

Women may age gracefully by adding these activities into their daily routines, preserving their health, vigor, and independence for many years.

THANK YOU PAGE

Thank you for selecting this book. Your support is really appreciated. Similarly, I am grateful for the purchase of this book. Your input is valuable; please share your ideas in a review. It serves as a reference for future improvements. Enjoy reading and utilizing it!

Workout planner which is suitable for taking record of progress

Weekly
Workout Planner

Week : _______________

Month: _______________

Sunday

Monday

Tuesday

Goals

Goals

Goals

Wednesday

Thursday

Friday

Goals

Goals

Goals

Saturday

Water Tracker

Goals

Mood

Motivation _______________

Weekly
Workout Planner

Week : ________________

Month: ________________

Sunday

Monday

Tuesday

Goals

Goals

Goals

Wednesday

Thursday

Friday

Goals

Goals

Goals

Saturday

Water Tracker

Goals

Mood

Motivation ________________________________

Weekly Workout Planner

Week: _______________

Month: _______________

Sunday

Goals

Monday

Goals

Tuesday

Goals

Wednesday

Goals

Thursday

Goals

Friday

Goals

Saturday

Goals

Water Tracker

Goals

Mood

Motivation _______________

Weekly Workout Planner

Week : __________________

Month: __________________

Sunday

Monday

Tuesday

Goals

Goals

Goals

Wednesday

Thursday

Friday

Goals

Goals

Goals

Saturday

Water Tracker

Goals

Mood

Motivation ______________________________

Weekly Workout Planner

Week : _______________

Month: _______________

Sunday

Monday

Tuesday

Goals

Goals

Goals

Wednesday

Thursday

Friday

Goals

Goals

Goals

Saturday

Water Tracker

Goals

Mood

Motivation _______________

Weekly Workout Planner

Week : ___________

Month: ___________

Sunday

Goals

Monday

Goals

Tuesday

Goals

Wednesday

Goals

Thursday

Goals

Friday

Goals

Saturday

Goals

Water Tracker

Mood

Motivation

Weekly Workout Planner

Week : ________________

Month: ________________

Sunday

Monday

Tuesday

Goals

Goals

Goals

Wednesday

Thursday

Friday

Goals

Goals

Goals

Saturday

Water Tracker

Goals

Mood

Motivation _______________________________

Weekly Workout Planner

Week : ___________

Month: ___________

Sunday

Goals

Monday

Goals

Tuesday

Goals

Wednesday

Goals

Thursday

Goals

Friday

Goals

Saturday

Goals

Water Tracker

Mood

Motivation ______________________________

Weekly

Workout Planner

Week: ___________

Month: ___________

Sunday	Monday	Tuesday
Goals	Goals	**Goals**

Wednesday	Thursday	Friday
Goals	**Goals**	Goals

Saturday	Water Tracker
Goals	**Mood**

Motivation ________________________

____

____

____

____

Weekly
Workout Planner

Week : ___________

Month: ___________

Sunday

Monday

Tuesday

Goals

Goals

Goals

Wednesday

Thursday

Friday

Goals

Goals

Goals

Saturday

Water Tracker

Goals

Mood

Motivation ________________________________

Weekly
Workout Planner

Week : ___________

Month: ___________

Sunday

Monday

Tuesday

Goals

Goals

Goals

Wednesday

Thursday

Friday

Goals

Goals

Goals

Saturday

Water Tracker

Goals

Mood

Motivation

Weekly
Workout Planner

Week: _______________

Month: _______________

Sunday	Monday	Tuesday
Goals	Goals	Goals

Wednesday	Thursday	Friday
Goals	Goals	Goals

Saturday

Water Tracker

Goals

Mood

Motivation _______________

Weekly Workout Planner

Week: _______________

Month: _______________

Sunday

Goals

Monday

Goals

Tuesday

Goals

Wednesday

Goals

Thursday

Goals

Friday

Goals

Saturday

Goals

Water Tracker

Goals

Mood

Motivation

Weekly
Workout Planner

Week : _______________

Month: _______________

Sunday	Monday	Tuesday
Goals	Goals	Goals

Wednesday	Thursday	Friday
Goals	Goals	Goals

Saturday

Goals

Water Tracker

Mood

Motivation

Weekly Workout Planner

Week: _______________

Month: _______________

Sunday	Monday	Tuesday
Goals	Goals	**Goals**

Wednesday	Thursday	Friday
Goals	**Goals**	Goals

Saturday	Water Tracker
Goals	**Mood** 😣 😁 🙂 😊 😞

Motivation _______________
____
____
____
____

Weekly
Workout Planner

Week : _______________

Month: _______________

Sunday

Monday

Tuesday

Goals

Goals

Goals

Wednesday

Thursday

Friday

Goals

Goals

Goals

Saturday

Water Tracker

Goals

Mood

Motivation _________________________

Weekly
Workout Planner

Week : ______________

Month: ______________

Sunday

Monday

Tuesday

Goals

Goals

Goals

Wednesday

Thursday

Friday

Goals

Goals

Goals

Saturday

Water Tracker

Goals

Mood

Motivation ________________________________

Weekly Workout Planner

Week: __________

Month: __________

Sunday

Goals

Monday

Goals

Tuesday

Goals

Wednesday

Goals

Thursday

Goals

Friday

Goals

Saturday

Goals

Water Tracker

Goals

Mood

Motivation ________________

Weekly Workout Planner

Week : _______________

Month: _______________

Sunday

Goals

Monday

Goals

Tuesday

Goals

Wednesday

Goals

Thursday

Goals

Friday

Goals

Saturday

Goals

Water Tracker

Mood

Motivation _______________________________

Weekly Workout Planner

Week : _______________

Month: _______________

Sunday	Monday	Tuesday
Goals	Goals	Goals

Wednesday	Thursday	Friday
Goals	Goals	Goals

Saturday	Water Tracker
Goals	

Mood

Motivation ____

____

____

____

Weekly Workout Planner

Week: ______________

Month: ______________

Sunday

Goals

Monday

Goals

Tuesday

Goals

Wednesday

Goals

Thursday

Goals

Friday

Goals

Saturday

Goals

Water Tracker

Mood

Motivation _________________________________

Weekly Workout Planner

Week: ___________

Month: ___________

Sunday

Goals

Monday

Goals

Tuesday

Goals

Wednesday

Goals

Thursday

Goals

Friday

Goals

Saturday

Goals

Water Tracker

Mood

Motivation ___________

Weekly
Workout Planner

Week : _______________

Month: _______________

Sunday

Monday

Tuesday

Goals

Goals

Goals

Wednesday

Thursday

Friday

Goals

Goals

Goals

Saturday

Water Tracker

Goals

Mood

Motivation _______________________________

Weekly Workout Planner

Week: ___________

Month: ___________

Sunday   Monday   Tuesday

Goals   Goals   Goals

Wednesday   Thursday   Friday

Goals   Goals   Goals

Saturday   Water Tracker

Goals   **Mood**

Motivation ________________________________

Weekly Workout Planner

Week: _____________

Month: _____________

Sunday	Monday	Tuesday
Goals	Goals	**Goals**

Wednesday	Thursday	Friday
Goals	**Goals**	Goals

Saturday

Water Tracker

Goals

Mood

Motivation __________________________

Weekly Workout Planner

Week: __________

Month: __________

Sunday

Goals

Monday

Goals

Tuesday

Goals

Wednesday

Goals

Thursday

Goals

Friday

Goals

Saturday

Goals

Water Tracker

Goals

Mood

Motivation _______________________________

Weekly Workout Planner

Week : ___________

Month: ___________

Sunday

Monday

Tuesday

Goals

Goals

Goals

Wednesday

Thursday

Friday

Goals

Goals

Goals

Saturday

Water Tracker

Goals

Mood

Motivation ___________________________

Weekly Workout Planner

Week: _______________

Month: _______________

Sunday

Monday

Tuesday

Goals

Goals

Goals

Wednesday

Thursday

Friday

Goals

Goals

Goals

Saturday

Water Tracker

Goals

Mood

Motivation ___________________________

Weekly Workout Planner

Week : _____________

Month: _____________

Sunday

Monday

Tuesday

Goals

Goals

Goals

Wednesday

Thursday

Friday

Goals

Goals

Goals

Saturday

Water Tracker

Goals

Mood

Motivation ________________________

Weekly Workout Planner

Week : _______________

Month: _______________

Sunday	Monday	Tuesday
Goals	Goals	Goals

Wednesday	Thursday	Friday
Goals	Goals	Goals

Saturday

Water Tracker

Goals

Mood

Motivation _______________

Weekly
Workout Planner

Week : _______________

Month: _______________

Sunday

Monday

Tuesday

Goals

Goals

Goals

Wednesday

Thursday

Friday

Goals

Goals

Goals

Saturday

Water Tracker

Goals

Mood

Motivation _______________

Weekly
Workout Planner

Week : _______________

Month: _______________

Sunday	Monday	Tuesday
Goals	Goals	Goals

Wednesday	Thursday	Friday
Goals	Goals	Goals

Saturday

Water Tracker

Goals

Mood

Motivation _______________

Weekly Workout Planner

Week : __________

Month: __________

Sunday	Monday	Tuesday
Goals	Goals	**Goals**

Wednesday	Thursday	Friday
Goals	**Goals**	Goals

Saturday	Water Tracker
Goals	**Mood**

Motivation ________________________________

Weekly Workout Planner

Week : __________

Month: __________

Sunday

Goals

Monday

Goals

Tuesday

Goals

Wednesday

Goals

Thursday

Goals

Friday

Goals

Saturday

Goals

Water Tracker

Goals

Mood

Motivation __________

Weekly
Workout Planner

Week : __________

Month: __________

Sunday

Monday

Tuesday

Goals

Goals

Goals

Wednesday

Thursday

Friday

Goals

Goals

Goals

Saturday

Water Tracker

Goals

Mood

Motivation

Weekly Workout Planner

Week: ___________

Month: ___________

Sunday

Goals

Monday

Goals

Tuesday

Goals

Wednesday

Goals

Thursday

Goals

Friday

Goals

Saturday

Goals

Water Tracker

Mood

Motivation ___________________________

Weekly Workout Planner

Week: _______________

Month: _______________

Sunday	Monday	Tuesday
Goals	Goals	Goals

Wednesday	Thursday	Friday
Goals	Goals	Goals

Saturday	Water Tracker
Goals	Mood

Mood

Motivation

____

____

____

____

Weekly
Workout Planner

Week : _______________

Month: _______________

Sunday

Monday

Tuesday

Goals

Goals

Goals

Wednesday

Thursday

Friday

Goals

Goals

Goals

Saturday

Water Tracker

Goals

Mood

Motivation _______________

Weekly Workout Planner

Week : _______________

Month: _______________

Sunday

Monday

Tuesday

Goals

Goals

Goals

Wednesday

Thursday

Friday

Goals

Goals

Goals

Saturday

Water Tracker

Goals

Mood

Motivation _______________

Weekly Workout Planner

Week : _______________

Month: _______________

Sunday

Goals

Monday

Goals

Tuesday

Goals

Wednesday

Goals

Thursday

Goals

Friday

Goals

Saturday

Goals

Water Tracker

Mood

Motivation _______________

____

Weekly Workout Planner

Week: _______________

Month: _______________

Sunday	Monday	Tuesday
Goals	Goals	Goals

Wednesday	Thursday	Friday
Goals	Goals	Goals

Saturday	Water Tracker
Goals	

Mood

😣 😁 😐 🙂 🙁

Motivation _______________________________
____
____
____
____

Weekly Workout Planner

Week: ________________

Month: ________________

Sunday

Goals

Monday

Goals

Tuesday

Goals

Wednesday

Goals

Thursday

Goals

Friday

Goals

Saturday

Goals

Water Tracker

Goals

Mood

Motivation ________________

Weekly Workout Planner

Week: ___________

Month: ___________

Sunday	Monday	Tuesday
Goals	Goals	**Goals**

Wednesday	Thursday	Friday
Goals	**Goals**	Goals

Saturday	Water Tracker
Goals	

Mood

😖 😁 😌 😊 😫

Motivation ________________________________

____

____

____

Weekly Workout Planner

Week: _____________

Month: _____________

Sunday

Goals

Monday

Goals

Tuesday

Goals

Wednesday

Goals

Thursday

Goals

Friday

Goals

Saturday

Goals

Water Tracker

Mood

Motivation _______________________

Weekly
Workout Planner

Week : _______________

Month: _______________

Sunday

Goals

Monday

Goals

Tuesday

Goals

Wednesday

Goals

Thursday

Goals

Friday

Goals

Saturday

Goals

Water Tracker

Goals

Mood

Motivation _________________________

Weekly Workout Planner

Week: _______________

Month: _______________

Sunday

Goals

Monday

Goals

Tuesday

Goals

Wednesday

Goals

Thursday

Goals

Friday

Goals

Saturday

Goals

Water Tracker

Goals

Mood

Motivation _______________

Weekly Workout Planner

Week: ___________

Month: ___________

Sunday	Monday	Tuesday
Goals	Goals	Goals

Wednesday	Thursday	Friday
Goals	Goals	Goals

Saturday	Water Tracker
Goals	

Mood

Motivation ____

____

____

____

____

Weekly Workout Planner

Week : ______________

Month: ______________

Sunday

Goals

Monday

Goals

Tuesday

Goals

Wednesday

Goals

Thursday

Goals

Friday

Goals

Saturday

Goals

Water Tracker

Goals

Mood

Motivation ________________________

Weekly Workout Planner

Week : _____________

Month: _____________

Sunday

Goals

Monday

Goals

Tuesday

Goals

Wednesday

Goals

Thursday

Goals

Friday

Goals

Saturday

Goals

Water Tracker

Mood

Motivation ________________________

Weekly
Workout Planner

Week : _____________

Month: _____________

Sunday

Monday

Tuesday

Goals

Goals

Goals

Wednesday

Thursday

Friday

Goals

Goals

Goals

Saturday

Water Tracker

Goals

Mood

Motivation _______________________

Weekly Workout Planner

Week: ______________

Month: ______________

Sunday

Monday

Tuesday

Goals

Goals

Goals

Wednesday

Thursday

Friday

Goals

Goals

Goals

Saturday

Water Tracker

Goals

Mood

Motivation ________________________________

Weekly Workout Planner

Week: ________________

Month: ________________

Sunday

Monday

Tuesday

Goals

Goals

Goals

Wednesday

Thursday

Friday

Goals

Goals

Goals

Saturday

Water Tracker

Goals

Mood

Motivation ________________________________

Weekly Workout Planner

Week: _______________

Month: _______________

Sunday	Monday	Tuesday
Goals	Goals	**Goals**

Wednesday	Thursday	Friday
Goals	**Goals**	Goals

Saturday

Water Tracker

Goals

Mood

Motivation _______________

Weekly
Workout Planner

Week: ___________

Month: ___________

Sunday | Monday | Tuesday

Goals | Goals | Goals

Wednesday | Thursday | Friday

Goals | Goals | Goals

Saturday | Water Tracker

Goals

Mood

Motivation ___________

Weekly
Workout Planner

Week : _______________

Month: _______________

Sunday	Monday	Tuesday
Goals	Goals	Goals

Wednesday	Thursday	Friday
Goals	Goals	Goals

Saturday

Goals

Water Tracker

Mood

Motivation ________________________

Weekly Workout Planner

Week : __________

Month: __________

Sunday

Monday

Tuesday

Goals

Goals

Goals

Wednesday

Thursday

Friday

Goals

Goals

Goals

Saturday

Water Tracker

Goals

Mood

Motivation __________

Weekly
Workout Planner

Week : ___________

Month: ___________

Sunday

Monday

Tuesday

Goals

Goals

Goals

Wednesday

Thursday

Friday

Goals

Goals

Goals

Saturday

Water Tracker

Goals

Mood

Motivation

Weekly Workout Planner

Week : _______________

Month: _______________

Sunday

Goals

Monday

Goals

Tuesday

Goals

Wednesday

Goals

Thursday

Goals

Friday

Goals

Saturday

Goals

Water Tracker

Mood

Motivation _______________

Weekly Workout Planner

Week : ______________

Month: ______________

Sunday

Goals

Monday

Goals

Tuesday

Goals

Wednesday

Goals

Thursday

Goals

Friday

Goals

Saturday

Goals

Water Tracker

Goals

Mood

Motivation

____

Weekly
Workout Planner

Week : _______________

Month: _______________

Sunday

Monday

Tuesday

Goals

Goals

Goals

Wednesday

Thursday

Friday

Goals

Goals

Goals

Saturday

Water Tracker

Goals

Mood

Motivation _______________

Weekly Workout Planner

Week: _______________

Month: _______________

Sunday

Goals

Monday

Goals

Tuesday

Goals

Wednesday

Goals

Thursday

Goals

Friday

Goals

Saturday

Goals

Water Tracker

Goals

Mood

Motivation _______________

Weekly
Workout Planner

Week : _______________

Month: _______________

Sunday

Monday

Tuesday

Goals

Goals

Goals

Wednesday

Thursday

Friday

Goals

Goals

Goals

Saturday

Water Tracker

Goals

Mood

Motivation _______________

Weekly
Workout Planner

Week : _______________

Month: _______________

Sunday	Monday	Tuesday
Goals	Goals	**Goals**

Wednesday	Thursday	Friday
Goals	**Goals**	Goals

Saturday   Water Tracker

Goals   **Mood**

Motivation _______________________________

Weekly
Workout Planner

Week : _______________

Month: _______________

Sunday

Monday

Tuesday

Goals

Goals

Goals

Wednesday

Thursday

Friday

Goals

Goals

Goals

Saturday

Water Tracker

Goals

Mood

Motivation _______________

Weekly
Workout Planner

Week : ________________

Month: ________________

Sunday	Monday	Tuesday
Goals	Goals	**Goals**

Wednesday	Thursday	Friday
Goals	**Goals**	Goals

Saturday	Water Tracker
Goals	

Mood

Motivation ________________

Weekly
Workout Planner

Week : _______________

Month: _______________

Sunday

Monday

Tuesday

Goals

Goals

Goals

Wednesday

Thursday

Friday

Goals

Goals

Goals

Saturday

Water Tracker

Goals

Mood

Motivation ________________________

Weekly Workout Planner

Week : ___________

Month: ___________

Sunday

Goals

Monday

Goals

Tuesday

Goals

Wednesday

Goals

Thursday

Goals

Friday

Goals

Saturday

Goals

Water Tracker

Goals

Mood

Motivation ________________________

Weekly
Workout Planner

Week : _______________

Month: _______________

Sunday

Monday

Tuesday

Goals

Goals

Goals

Wednesday

Thursday

Friday

Goals

Goals

Goals

Saturday

Water Tracker

Goals

Mood

Motivation _______________________

Weekly
Workout Planner

Week : _______________

Month: _______________

Sunday	Monday	Tuesday
Goals	Goals	**Goals**

Wednesday	Thursday	Friday
Goals	**Goals**	Goals

Saturday	Water Tracker
Goals	**Mood**

Mood

Motivation ______________________

Weekly
Workout Planner

Week : ________________

Month: ________________

Sunday

Monday

Tuesday

Goals

Goals

Goals

Wednesday

Thursday

Friday

Goals

Goals

Goals

Saturday

Water Tracker

Goals

Mood

Motivation ________________

Weekly
Workout Planner

Week : _______________

Month: _______________

Sunday

Monday

Tuesday

Goals

Goals

Goals

Wednesday

Thursday

Friday

Goals

Goals

Goals

Saturday

Water Tracker

Goals

Mood

Motivation ______________________________

Weekly Workout Planner

Week : _______________

Month: _______________

Sunday	Monday	Tuesday
Goals	Goals	Goals

Wednesday	Thursday	Friday
Goals	Goals	Goals

Saturday

Goals

Water Tracker

Mood

Motivation _______________

Weekly
Workout Planner

Week : _______________

Month: _______________

Sunday

Monday

Tuesday

Goals

Goals

Goals

Wednesday

Thursday

Friday

Goals

Goals

Goals

Saturday

Water Tracker

Goals

Mood

Motivation ______________________

Weekly Workout Planner

Week : ___________

Month: ___________

Sunday

Monday

Tuesday

Goals

Goals

Goals

Wednesday

Thursday

Friday

Goals

Goals

Goals

Saturday

Water Tracker

Goals

Mood

Motivation ______________________

Weekly
Workout Planner

Week : __________

Month: __________

Sunday

Monday

Tuesday

Goals

Goals

Goals

Wednesday

Thursday

Friday

Goals

Goals

Goals

Saturday

Water Tracker

Goals

Mood

Motivation

Weekly Workout Planner

Week : _______________

Month: _______________

Sunday

Goals

Monday

Goals

Tuesday

Goals

Wednesday

Goals

Thursday

Goals

Friday

Goals

Saturday

Goals

Water Tracker

Goals

Mood

Motivation _______________________________________

Weekly Workout Planner

Week : _______________

Month: _______________

Sunday

Monday

Tuesday

Goals

Goals

Goals

Wednesday

Thursday

Friday

Goals

Goals

Goals

Saturday

Water Tracker

Goals

Mood

Motivation _______________________________

Weekly
Workout Planner

Week : _______________

Month: _______________

Sunday

Monday

Tuesday

Goals

Goals

Goals

Wednesday

Thursday

Friday

Goals

Goals

Goals

Saturday

Water Tracker

Goals

Mood

Motivation _______________

Weekly Workout Planner

Week : _______________

Month: _______________

Sunday

Monday

Tuesday

Goals

Goals

Goals

Wednesday

Thursday

Friday

Goals

Goals

Goals

Saturday

Water Tracker

Goals

Mood

Motivation

Weekly
Workout Planner

Week : _______________

Month: _______________

Sunday

Monday

Tuesday

Goals

Goals

Goals

Wednesday

Thursday

Friday

Goals

Goals

Goals

Saturday

Water Tracker

Goals

Mood

Motivation _______________________________

Weekly Workout Planner

Week: _______________

Month: _______________

Sunday

Monday

Tuesday

Goals

Goals

Goals

Wednesday

Thursday

Friday

Goals

Goals

Goals

Saturday

Water Tracker

Goals

Mood

Motivation _______________

www.ingramcontent.com/pod-product-compliance
Lightning Source LLC
Chambersburg PA
CBHW050809260726
48660CB00004B/1334